JUICING RECIPES FOR PCOS

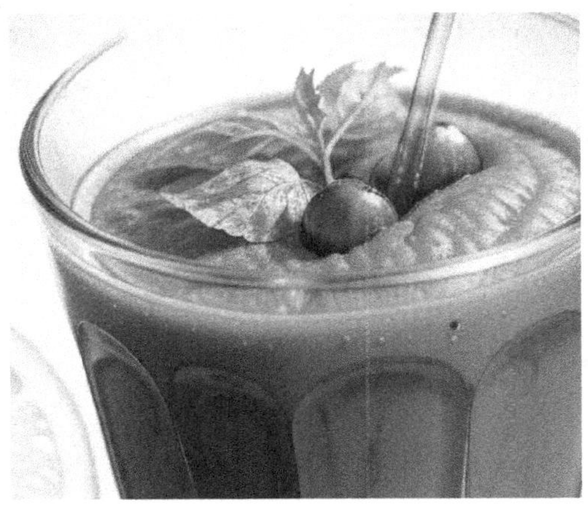

Boost your Health Naturally

JESSICA MURRAY

Dear Reader,

Thank you for the purchase. I hope you enjoy and love it, would you consider dropping an honest feedback/review, I will appreciate that and you can contact me using JessicaMurrayDietHelp@gmail.com if you have any questions, I will gladly respond

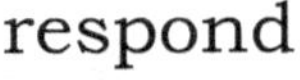

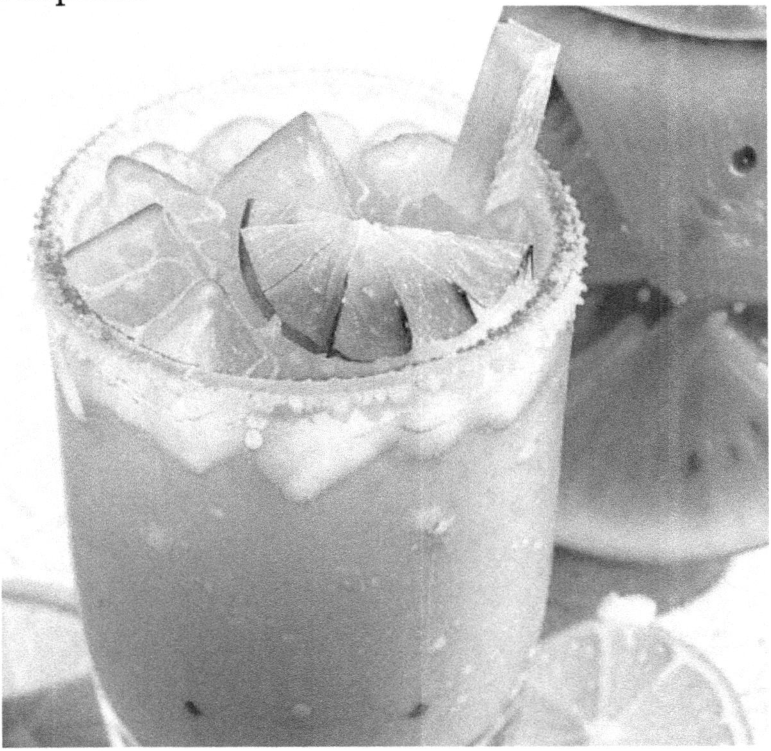

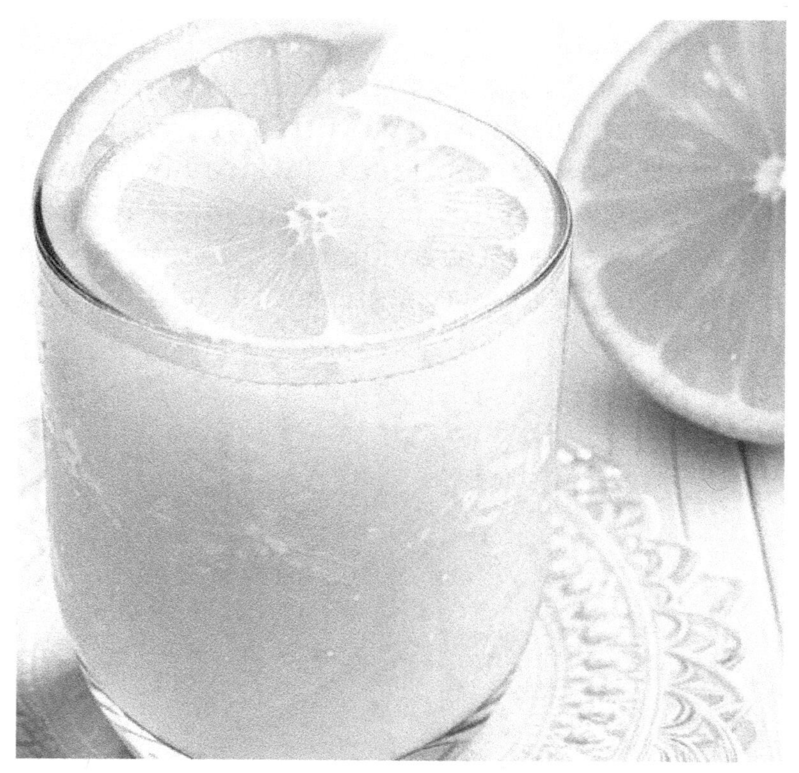

Table of Contents

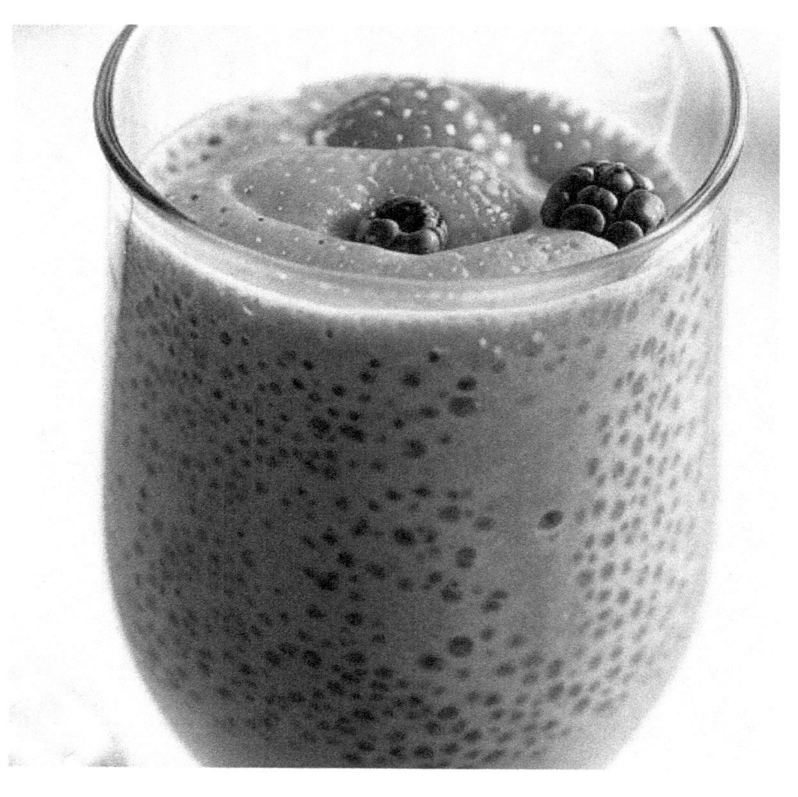

INTRODUCTION TO JUICING FOR PCOS

Imagine Emily, a lively woman who resides in the centre of the busy metropolis. She had ambitions and plans, but her fight with PCOS (Polycystic Ovary Syndrome) had turned into a never-ending struggle, dimming her aspirations. Her feelings of helplessness and defeat were brought on by the weight increase, mood changes, and irregular cycles.

She once happened to see a book named "Juicing for PCOS" while perusing the racks at a nearby bookstore. She took it up out of curiosity since it offered the possibility of a natural remedy for her persistent health issues.

Emily perused the book's pages, absorbing up information about how particular fruits, vegetables, and herbs could help with PCOS symptom management. She found new hope in the thorough explanations and colourful recipes. She made the decision to give it a try and started her transformational adventure.

Emily began her daily practice of making vibrant, nutrient-rich juices with a blender and fresh fruits. Knowing that she was nourishing her body from the inside out, she enjoyed every drink. She noticed changes as the vivacious energy of the fruits and veggies seemed to permeate her being.

Weeks moved into months, and Emily's life's before-and-after was nothing short of amazing. Her previously irregular periods started to become more predictable, and the additional weight she had been carrying for so long started to dissipate.

The internal change, which came from taking control of her health, was the most astounding transformation, though. She had not only discovered a cure for her PCOS, but also a road to healing and self-discovery.

Emily couldn't help but spread her accomplishment as she accepted her journey. Her enthusiasm spread quickly around her circle because it was contagious. Her narrative served as an inspiration to friends and acquaintances who began their own juicing journeys in search of their own "before-and-after".

So, my friend, if you find yourself faced with health obstacles, keep Emily's story in mind. Think about the prospect of your own amazing "before and after," propelled by the potential for healing from "Juicing for PCOS." You have a journey ahead of you, and each sip you take could bring you that much closer to your own brilliant metamorphosis.

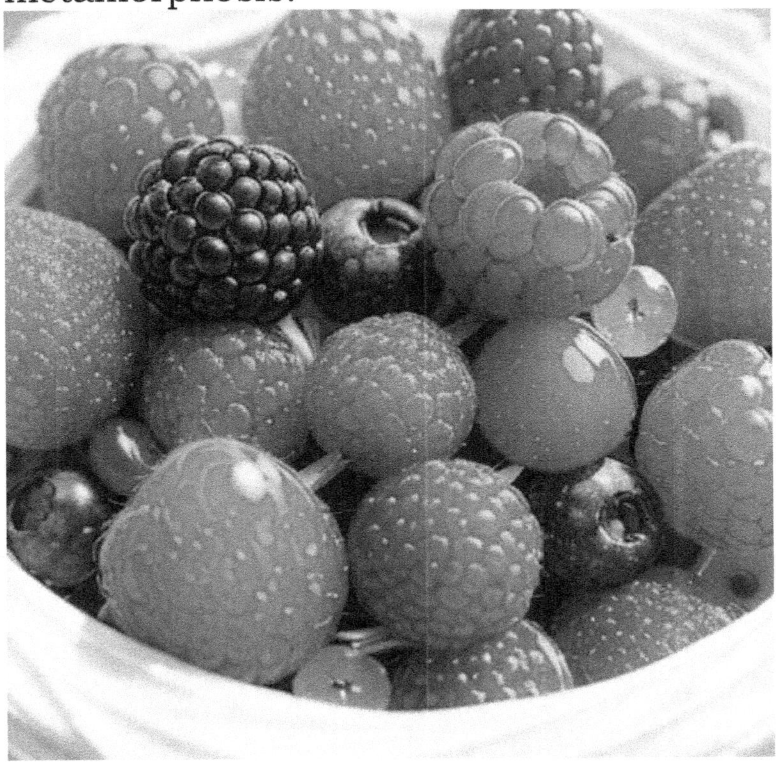

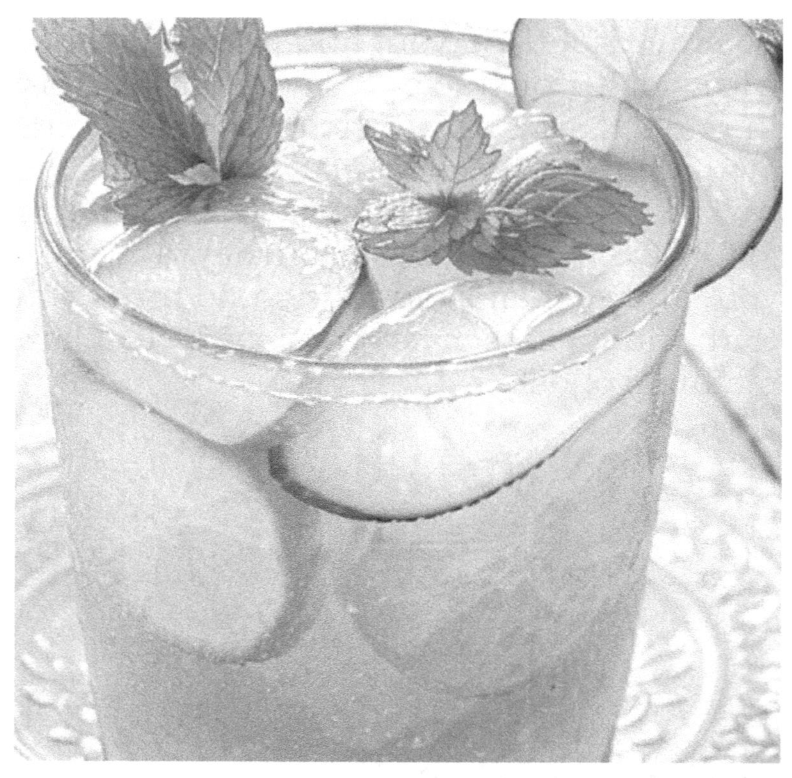

CHAPTER 1

Benefits Of Juicing For PCOS

Juicing offers potential benefits for individuals dealing with Polycystic Ovary Syndrome (PCOS). By incorporating fresh, nutrient-rich juices into their diet, PCOS sufferers may experience improved hormonal balance and symptom management. These vibrant concoctions provide a concentrated dose of vitamins, minerals, and antioxidants, aiding in regulating insulin levels and supporting weight management, both critical for PCOS management. Juices rich in dark leafy greens, like kale and spinach, can help combat inflammation and reduce oxidative stress, common issues in PCOS. Moreover, juicing can enhance digestion and gut health, positively impacting hormonal harmony. However, it's important to balance juices with whole foods to ensure adequate fibre intake and prevent blood sugar spikes. Consulting a healthcare provider or dietitian is advised to tailor juicing practices to individual needs and optimize the potential benefits for PCOS management

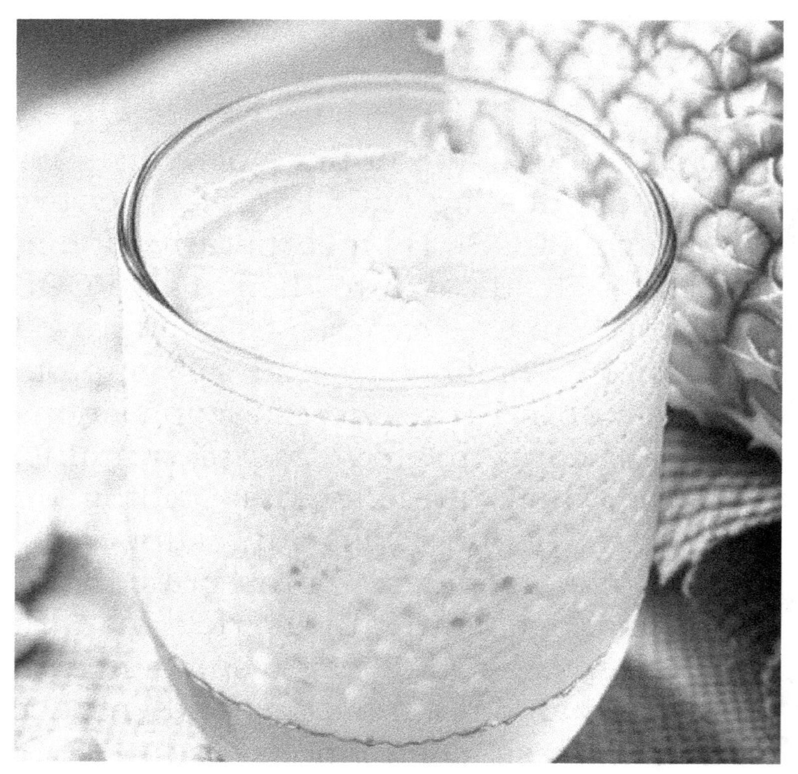

CHAPTER 2
Delicious Juicing Recipes For PCOS
Hormone-Balancing Green Juice

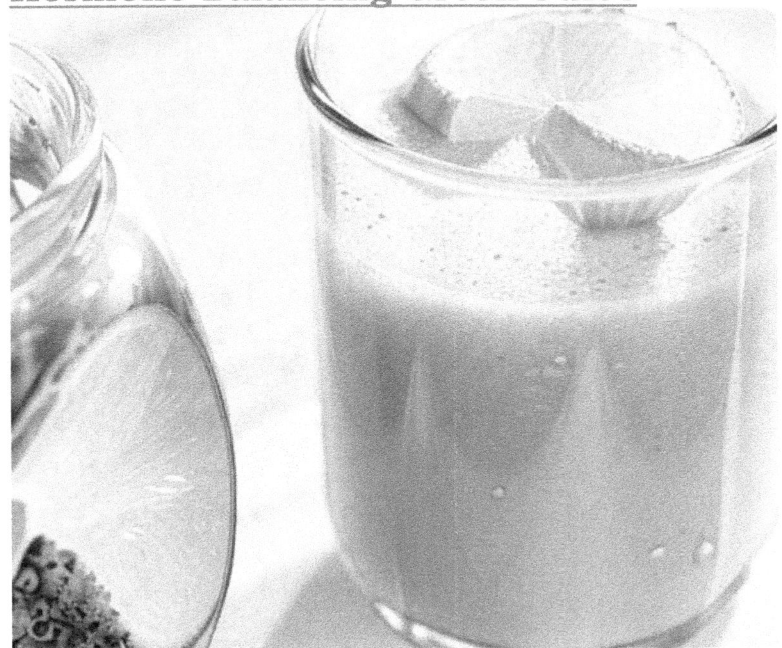

INGREDIENTS:
- two handfuls of spinach and
- one stalk of celery
- half a cucumber
- apples, two
- 1/2 lemon
- two fresh sprigs of parsley

INSTRUCTION:

- Thoroughly wash each component.
- Use a juicer to juice all the ingredients then serve right away.

Berry Bliss Antioxidant Blend

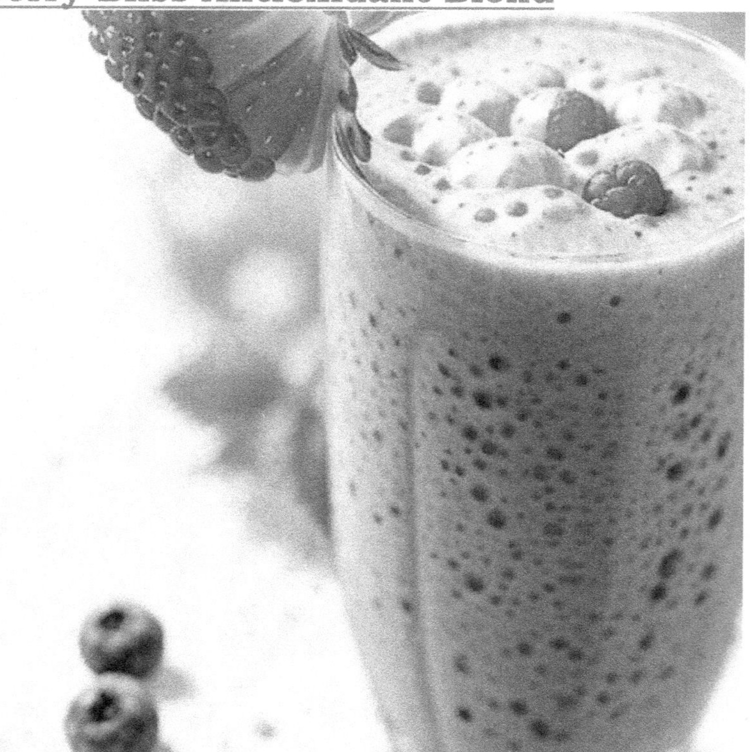

INGREDIENTS:
- 1/2 cup blueberries
- half a cup of strawberries
- Blackberries, 1/2 cup
- 1/four cup of raspberries

- 1/4 cup optional honey

INSTRUCTION:
- In a blender, combine all of the berries.
- Blend until smooth on high.
- If using honey, add it now and mix for a further 30 seconds.
- Either serve right away or keep chilled for up to 24 hours.

Citrus Delight for Insulin Sensitivity

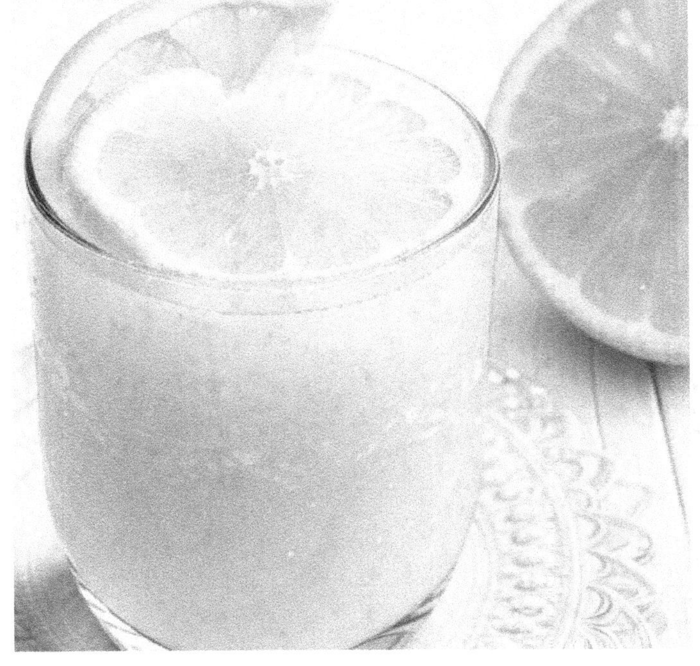

INGREDIENTS:

- Two teaspoons of freshly squeezed orange juice are the ingredients
- freshly squeezed lemon juice, two tablespoons
- 2 tablespoons grapefruit juice that has just been squeezed
- 1 teaspoon (optional) raw honey

INSTRUCTION:

- In a small bowl, combine the citrus liquids all together.
- If desired, stir in the honey.
- Immediately take a sip.

Gut-Healing Fibre Booster

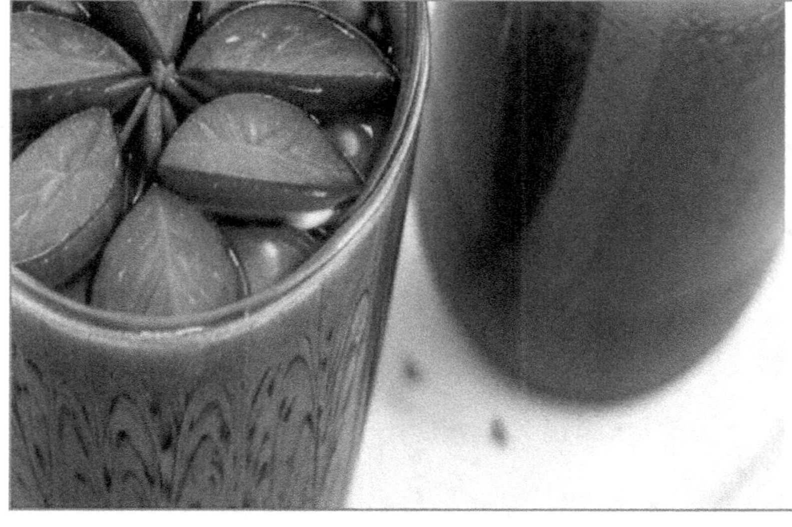

INGREDIENTS:
- 1/2 cup of ground flax seeds and 1/2 cup of oat bran
- psyllium husk powder, 1/4 cup
- 1 teaspoon of ginger, ground

INSTRUCTION:
- In a medium-sized bowl, mix together all of the necessary ingredients: in order to create the desired recipe.
- Combine by stirring.
- Either serve right away or keep for up to a month in an airtight container.

Energy-Boosting Beet Elixir

INGREDIENTS:
- 1 small beet, peeled and diced;
- 1/2 cup chunks of frozen mango;
- 1/2 cup pineapple chunks, frozen
- one cup of coconut water
- 1 teaspoon optional honey

INSTRUCTION:
- Place every ingredient in a blender.
- Blend until smooth on high.
- If using honey, add it now and mix for a further 30 seconds.
- Serve right away.

Anti-Inflammatory Turmeric Tonic

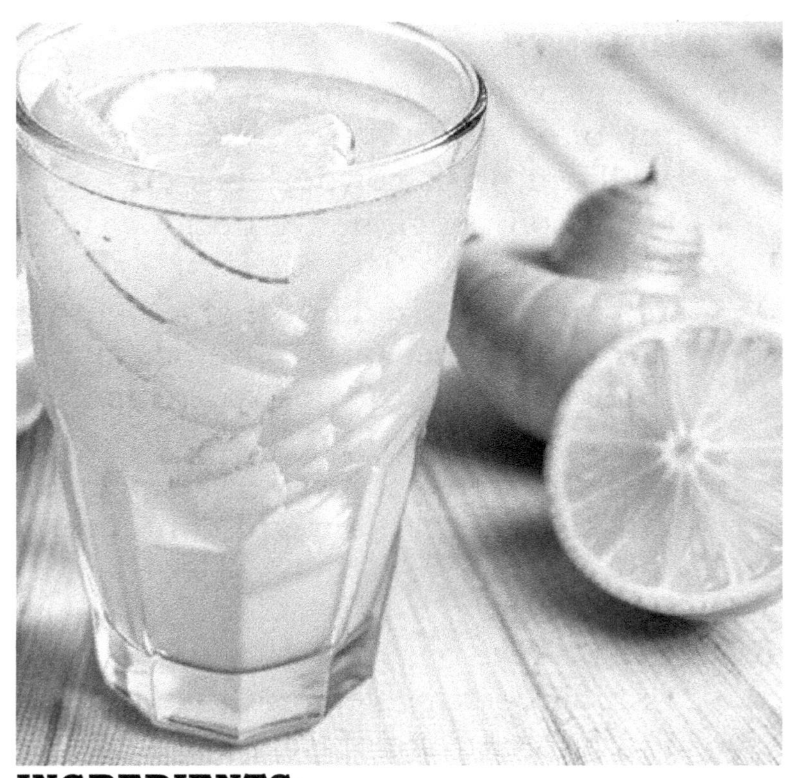

INGREDIENTS:

- One cup of freshly squeezed orange juice,
- one teaspoon of freshly grated turmeric root,
- one teaspoon of freshly ground ginger, and one teaspoon of freshly squeezed lemon juice 1 teaspoon (optional) raw honey

INSTRUCTION:

- In a medium-sized bowl, mix together all of the necessary ingredients: until they are completely incorporated.
- Combine by stirring.
- Either serve right away or keep chilled for up to 24 hours.

Leafy Greens and Flax Supercharge

INGREDIENTS:

- 2 cups fresh spinach, 2 cups fresh kale, and 1/4 cup ground flax seeds.
- 1/4 cup chopped raw almonds, 1 tablespoon olive oil

INSTRUCTION:

- In a medium bowl, mix the spinach, kale, flax seeds, and almonds.
- Add a drizzle of olive oil and blend by tossing.
- Serve right away.

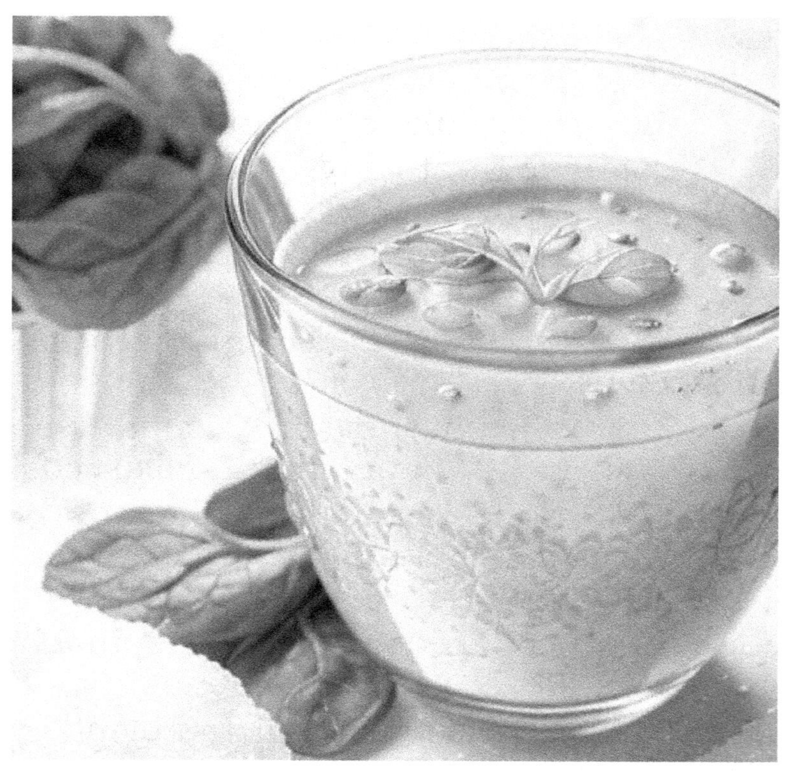

CHAPTER 3

Breakfast Recipes

Green Goddess Mix

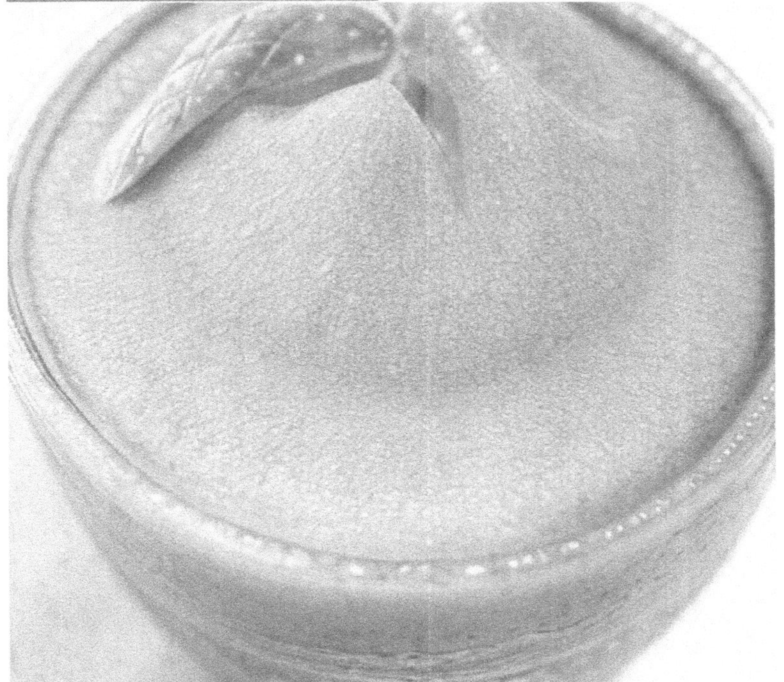

INGREDIENTS:

- 1 tablespoon fresh cilantro and 1/2 cup fresh parsley
- 1/four cup of fresh mint
- 25% of fresh basil
- Lemon juice, 1/4 cup
- Olive oil, two tablespoons
- 50 ml of sea salt

INSTRUCTION:

- Fill a blender or food processor with all the ingredients
- Blend and smooth the contents in a blender.
- To make sure all ingredients are pureed, occasionally scrape down the container's sides.
- Refrigerate for up to a week before serving

Berry Bliss Smoothie

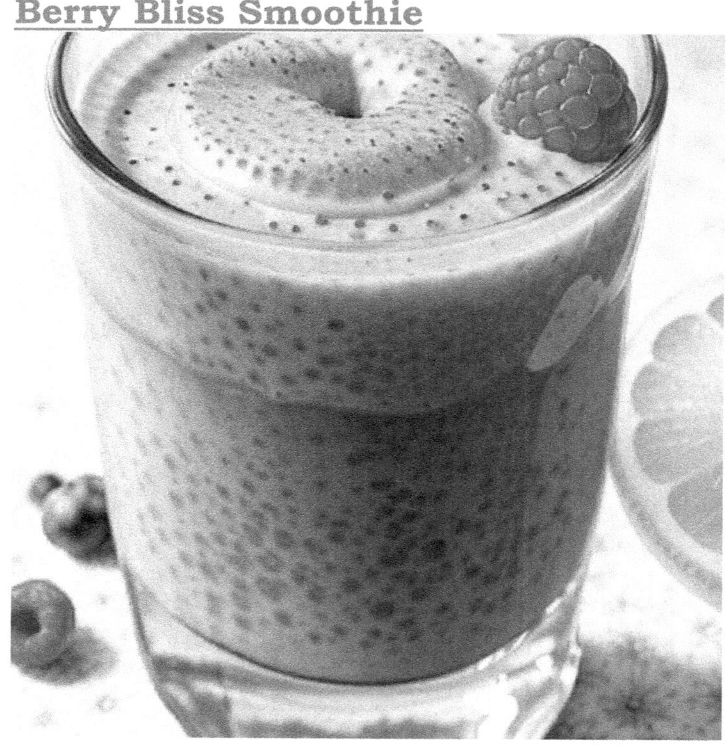

INGREDIENTS:

- 1 cup of mixed berries, either fresh or frozen
- one banana
- 0.5 cups of milk
- Greek yogurt, plain, in 1/2 cup
- Chia seeds, one tablespoon
- honey, 2 teaspoons

INSTRUCTION:

- Place all the ingredients in a blender, and process until thoroughly combined.
- Taste the dish and make any necessary flavour adjustments, such as adding more honey for sweetness or extra yogurt for smoothness.
- Pour the mixture into glasses and serve right away.

Citrus Delight Juice

INGREDIENTS:

- 1 grapefruit, chopped
- two oranges.
- 1 lemon
- 1 lime
- Honey, 1/4 cup
- 2-cups of water

INSTRUCTION:

- Peel and juice the lime, lemon, orange, and grapefruit.
- Strain the juice, then mix in the water and honey.
- Combine by stirring.
- Pour into cups, then take a sip.

Pineapple Turmeric Elixir

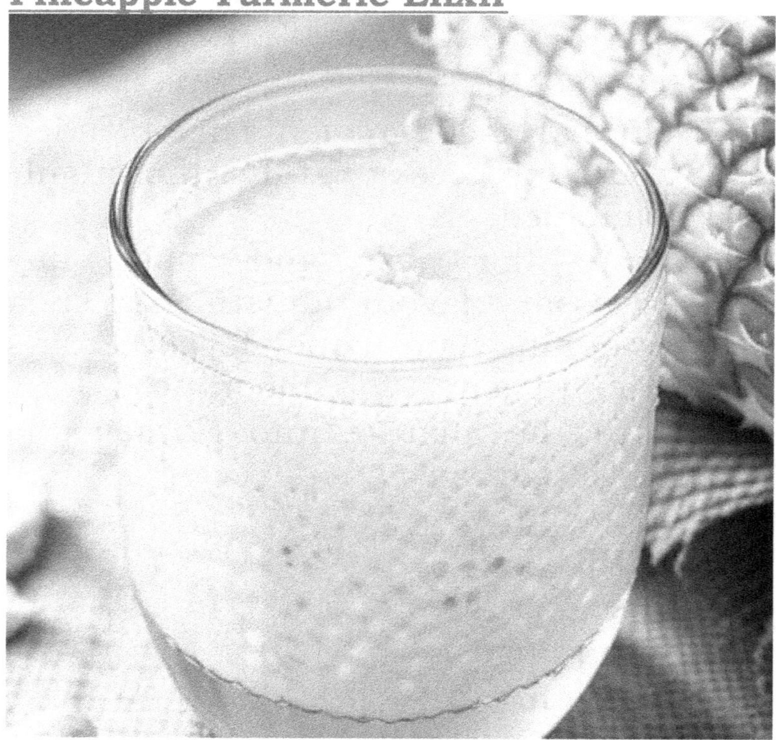

INGREDIENTS:

- 1 pineapple cup
- Turmeric, 1 teaspoon
- 1/8 teaspoon of ginger root

- 1/8 teaspoon cinnamon powder
- honey, 2 teaspoons
- Coconut water, 1 cup

INSTRUCTION:
- Place all the ingredients in a blender, and process until thoroughly combined.
- Add extra honey for sweetness and taste; adjust flavour as necessary.
- Pour into cups, then take a sip.

Beetroot Beauty Juice

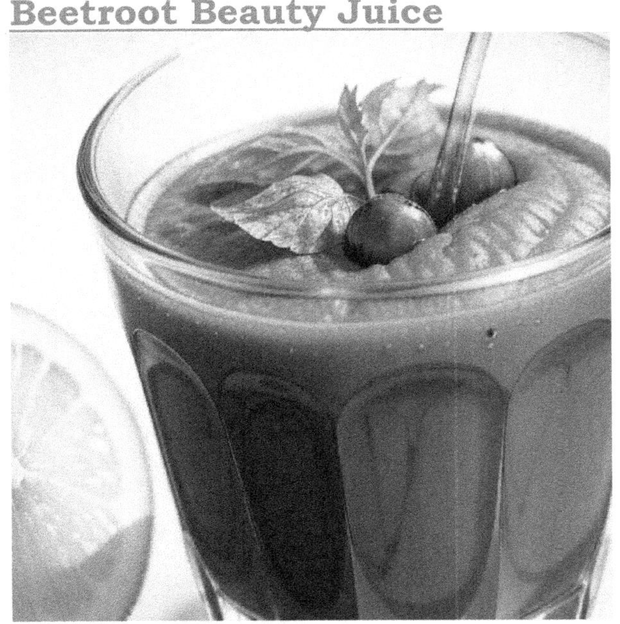

INGREDIENTS:
- 1 sizable beet

- One big carrot
- Celery stalks, two
- 50% of a lemon (with peel)
- Honey, two tablespoons
- 2-cups of water

INSTRUCTION:
- Peel the lemon, carrot, and beetroot.
- After juicing all the ingredients strain them.
- Combine water and honey by stirring.
- Pour into cups, then take a sip.

CHAPTER 4
Lunch Recipes
Cucumber Mint Refresher

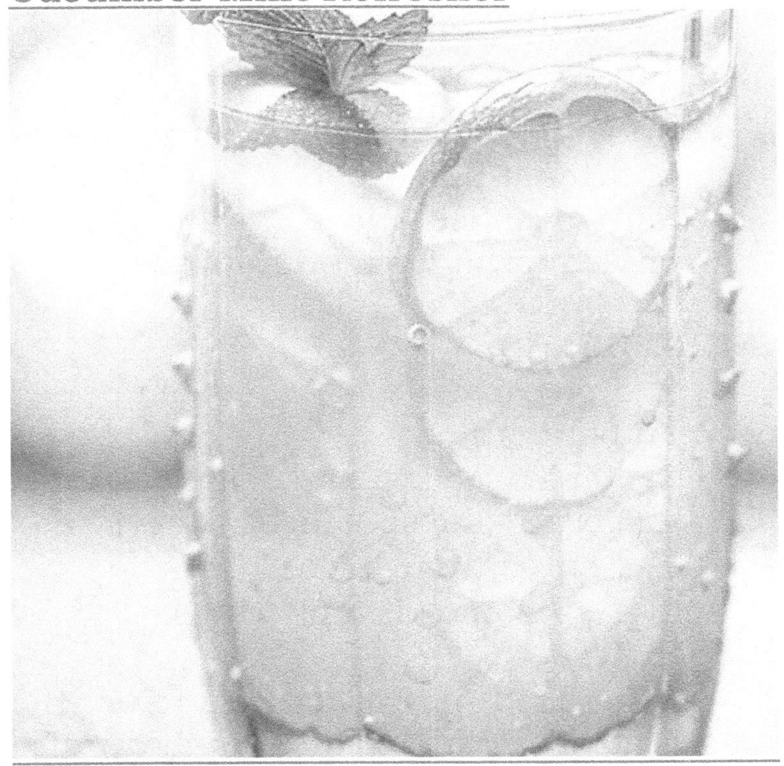

INGREDIENTS:

- 2 big cucumbers
- A half cup of fresh mint
- lime juice, 3/4 cup
- 2 agave nectar tablespoons
- 2 cups water

INSTRUCTION:
- Cut the cucumbers into pieces.
- In a food processor, combine the cucumbers, mint, lime juice, and agave nectar and process until smooth.
- Add water to the mixture after pouring it into a pitcher.
- Pour over ice and drink after being chilled for at least 30 minutes.

Carrot Ginger Zing

INGREDIENTS:
- 2 large carrots that have been peeled and grated;
- 2 tablespoons of freshly grated ginger; 2 tablespoons of honey;
- 1/4 cup orange juice.
- 2 glasses of sparkling water

INSTRUCTION:
- In a food processor, combine the grated carrots and ginger and pulse until smooth.
- Blend the honey and orange juice completely after adding them.
- Fill a pitcher with sparkling water after pouring the mixture into it.

- Pour over ice and drink after being chilled for at least 30 minutes.

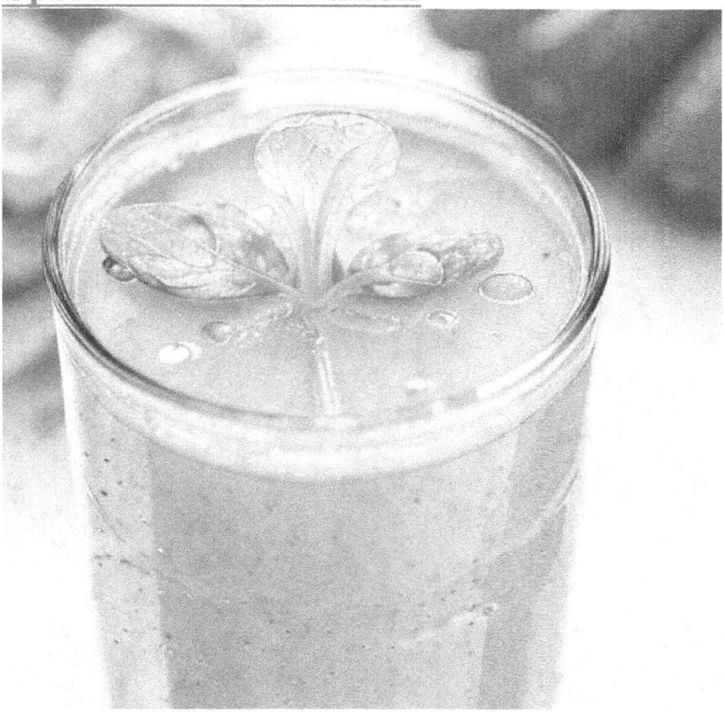

INGREDIENTS:

- 2 cups spinach and 1/4 cup freshly squeezed lemon juice
- 1/4 cup ground cinnamon and 1/4 cup honey
- 1/8 teaspoon freshly grated nutmeg
- 2 glasses of sparkling water

INSTRUCTION:

- In a food processor, combine the spinach, lemon juice, honey, cinnamon, and nutmeg. Process until smooth.
- Fill a pitcher with sparkling water after pouring the mixture into it.
- Pour over ice and drink after being chilled for at least 30 minutes.

Blueberry Spinach Fusion

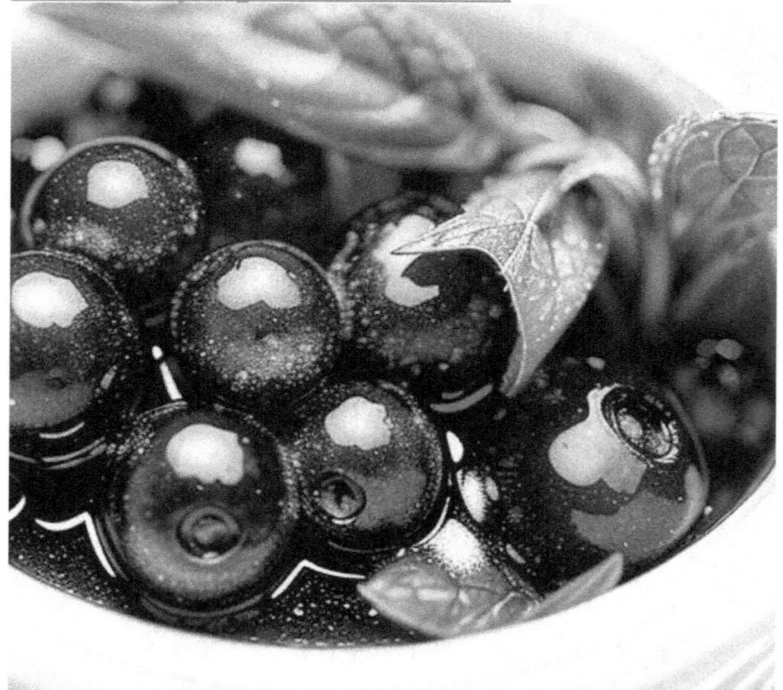

INGREDIENTS:

- 1 cup of fresh blueberries and 2 cups of spinach.
- 2 tablespoons of freshly squeezed lemon juice
- 1/4 cup of honey
- 2 glasses of sparkling water

INSTRUCTION:

- In a food processor, combine the spinach, blueberries, honey, and lemon juice and pulse until smooth.
- Fill a pitcher with sparkling water after pouring the mixture into it.
- Pour over ice and drink after being chilled for at least 30 minutes.

Kale Pineapple Pleasure

INGREDIENTS:

- 1 cup diced fresh pineapple and 2 cups greens.
- 2 tablespoons of honey
- 2 tablespoons of lime juice that has just been squeezed
- 2 glasses of sparkling water

INSTRUCTION:

- In a food processor, mix the kale, pineapple, honey, and lime juice until smooth.

- Fill a pitcher with sparkling water after pouring the mixture into it.
- Pour over ice and drink after being chilled for at least 30 minutes.

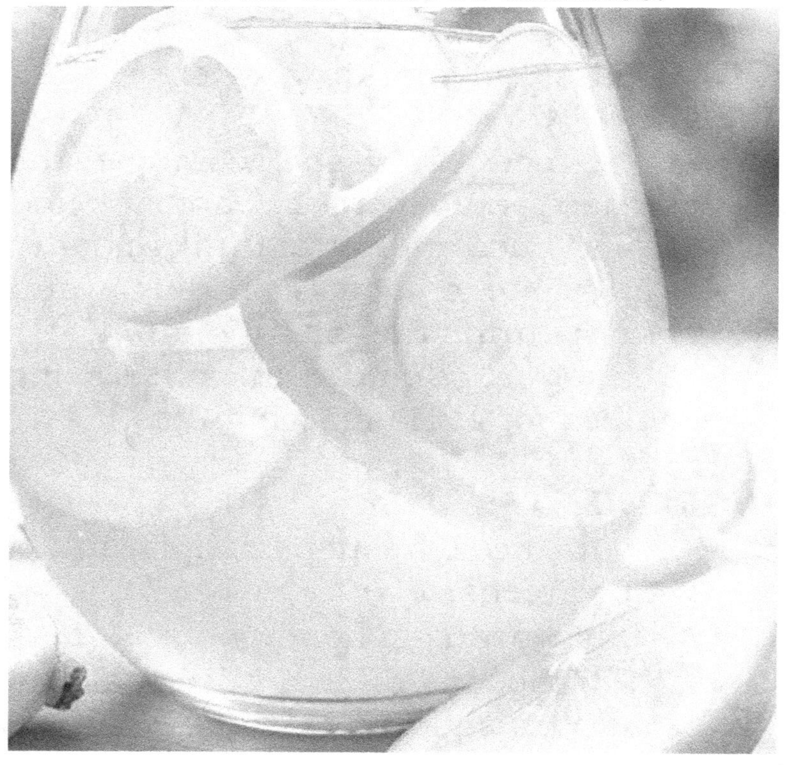

Dinner Recipes

Apple Cinnamon Sensation

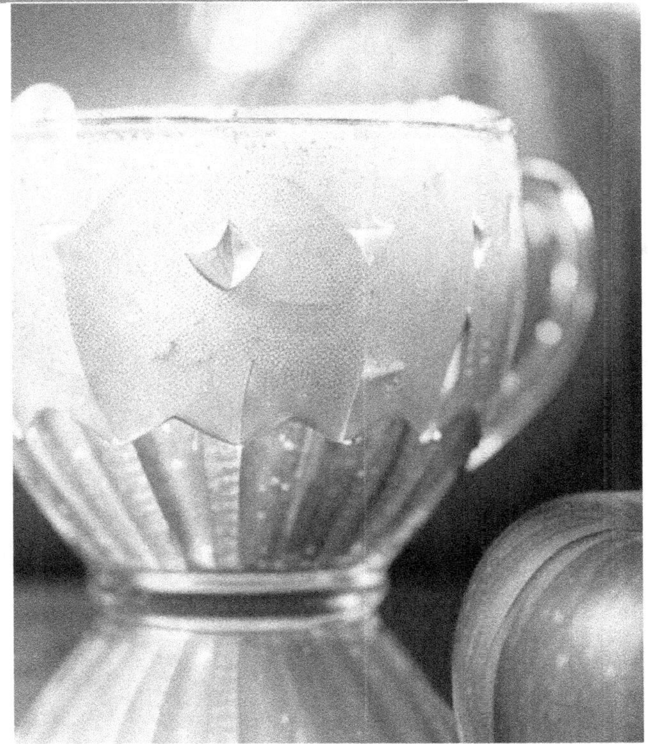

INGREDIENTS:

- 1 cored and sliced apple
- 1 teaspoon of cinnamon, ground
- a single cup of cold water
- optional sugar, honey, or maple syrup

INSTRUCTION:

- Add the apples to a blender and process until completely smooth.
- Blend together the cinnamon, water, and sweetener (if using).
- Serve chilled or on top of ice.

Papaya Passion Juice

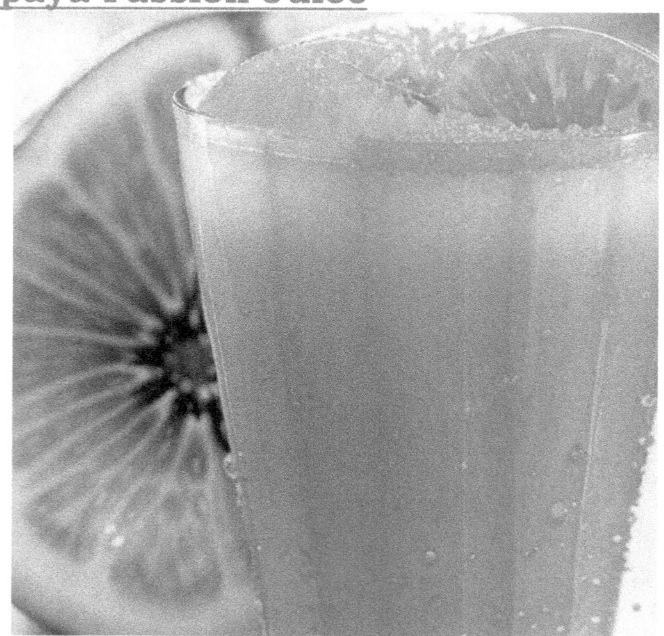

INGREDIENTS:

- 1 diced ripe papaya; 1/2 cup fresh or
- frozen pineapple; and 1/2 juiced lime
- two honey teaspoons and one cup of iced water

INSTRUCTION:

- Add all of the ingredients to a blender, and process until thoroughly combined.
- Pour over ice or serve chilled.

Watermelon Cooler

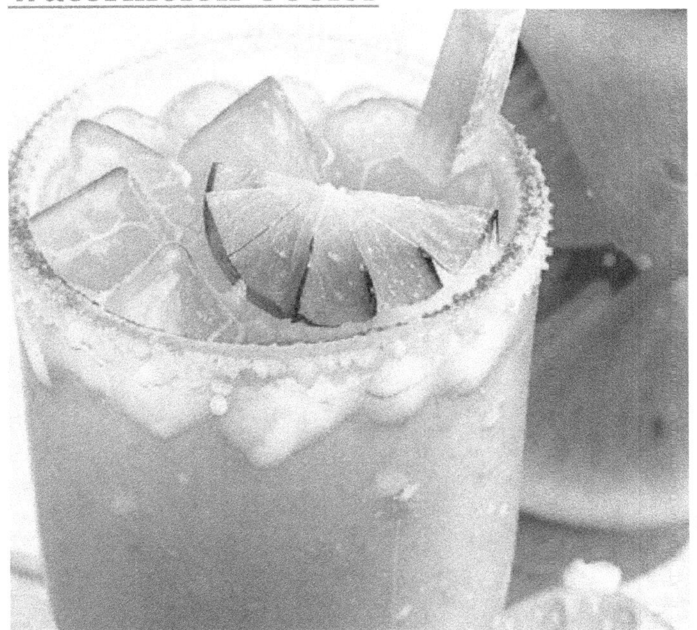

INGREDIENTS:

- three cups of chopped watermelon and half a lime.
- fresh mint leaves, 1/4 cup
- two cups of icy water
- Agar syrup or honey (optional)

INSTRUCTION:

- In order to make a smooth mixture of all the ingredients pour them into a blender and process them until they have been blended together completely.
- Add the sweetener (if using) and mix well.
- Serve chilled or on top of ice.

Mixed Berry Medley

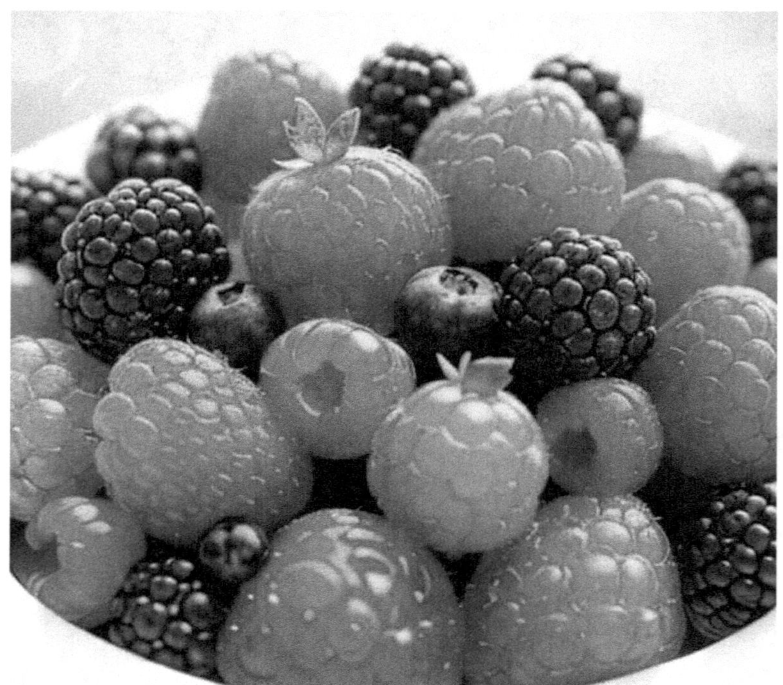

INGREDIENTS:

- 1/2 cup of strawberries, either fresh or frozen.
- 1/2 cup of blueberries, either fresh or frozen

INSTRUCTION:
- Add all of the ingredients to a blender, and process until thoroughly combined.
- Add the sweetener (if using) and mix well.
- Serve chilled or on top of ice.

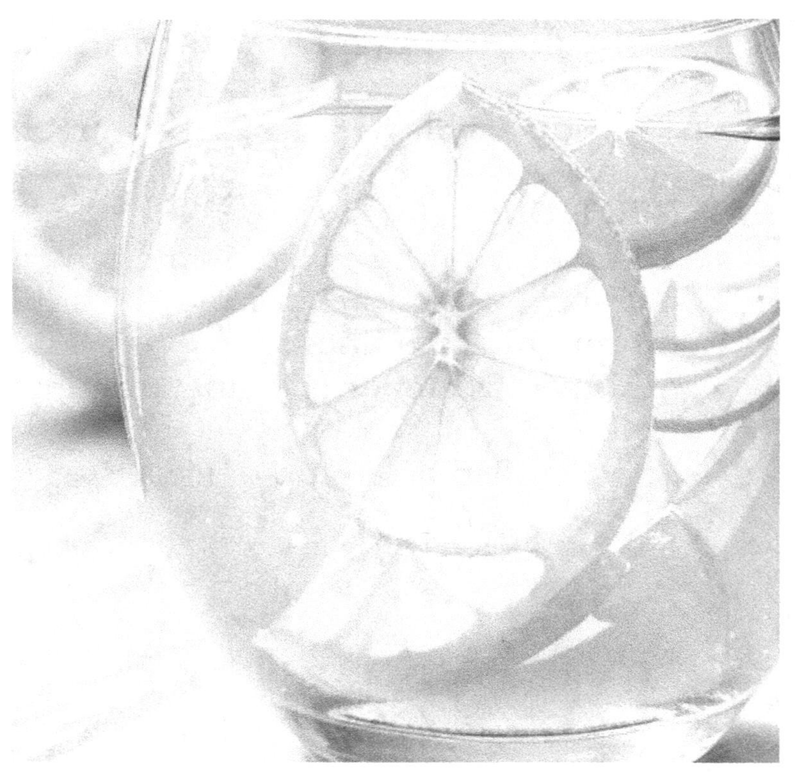

CONCLUSION

We've set out on a journey of renewal and empowerment within the pages of this book of PCOS juicing recipes. Each cuisine is a testament to the curative power of nature, from colourful fruits to nutrient-rich veggies. Remember that you have the ability to take care of your body, balance your hormones, and regain your vigour as you sip on these vibrant mixtures. Let these drinks serve as a source of motivation, pointing you in the direction of a healthy, energised life. May these recipes serve as your guides on the way to a better, happier you, and may your journey to healing be one of hope.

I'm grateful that you took the time to read my book. I hope you like it and it gave you something to think about. Thank You

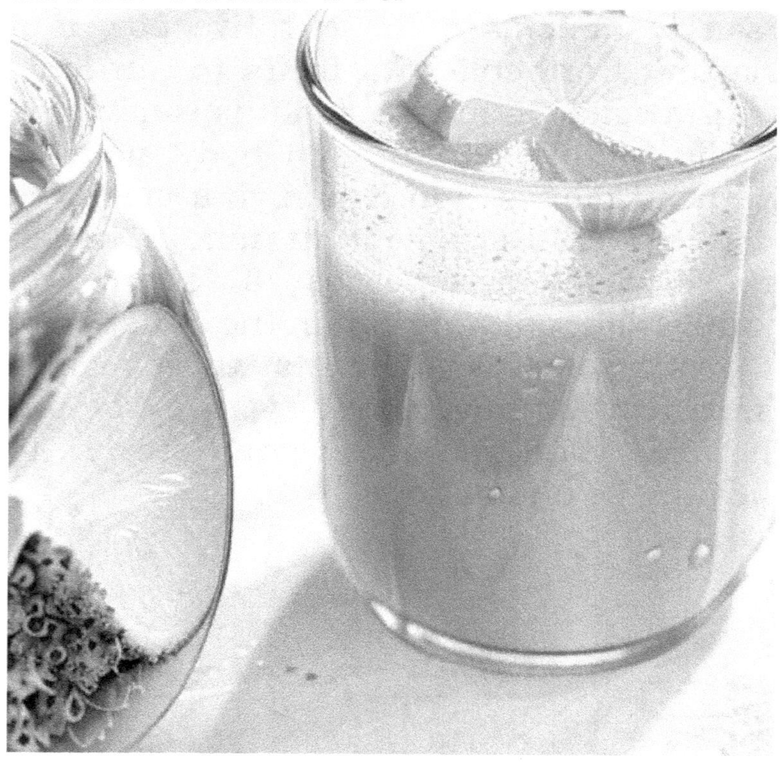

Weekly Meal Planner

KEY

B-Breakfast
L-Lunch
D-Dinner

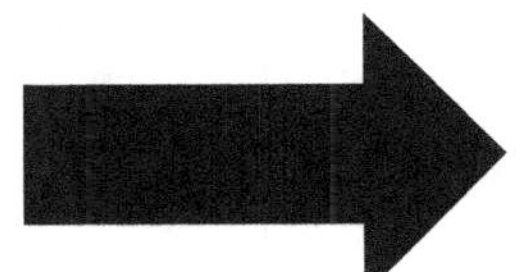

MONDAY	B	
	L	
	D	
TUESDAY	B	
	L	
	D	
WENESDAY	B	
	L	
	D	
THURSDAY	B	
	L	
	D	
FRIDAY	B	
	L	
	D	
SATURDAY	B	
	L	
	D	
SUNDAY	B	
	L	
	D	

MONDAY	B
	L
	D
TUESDAY	B
	L
	D
WENESDAY	B
	L
	D
THURSDAY	B
	L
	D
FRIDAY	B
	L
	D
SATURDAY	B
	L
	D
SUNDAY	B
	L
	D

MONDAY	B
	L
	D

TUESDAY	B
	L
	D

WENESDAY	B
	L
	D

THURSDAY	B
	L
	D

FRIDAY	B
	L
	D

SATURDAY	B
	L
	D

SUNDAY	B
	L
	D

MONDAY	B L D	
TUESDAY	B L D	
WENESDAY	B L D	
THURSDAY	B L D	
FRIDAY	B L D	
SATURDAY	B L D	
SUNDAY	B L D	

MONDAY	B
	L
	D

TUESDAY	B
	L
	D

WENESDAY	B
	L
	D

THURSDAY	B
	L
	D

FRIDAY	B
	L
	D

SATURDAY	B
	L
	D

SUNDAY	B
	L
	D

MONDAY	B
	L
	D

TUESDAY	B
	L
	D

WENESDAY	B
	L
	D

THURSDAY	B
	L
	D

FRIDAY	B
	L
	D

SATURDAY	B
	L
	D

SUNDAY	B
	L
	D

MONDAY	B
	L
	D
TUESDAY	B
	L
	D
WENESDAY	B
	L
	D
THURSDAY	B
	L
	D
FRIDAY	B
	L
	D
SATURDAY	B
	L
	D
SUNDAY	B
	L
	D

DAILY MEAL PLANNER

TO DO	
1	
2	
3	
4	
5	
6	
7	
8	
9	
10	

EXERCISE

GOAL ACTIVITIES

- ☐
- ☐
- ☐
- ☐
- ☐
- ☐
- ☐

SHOPPING

<table>
<tr><td colspan="2" align="center">MEALS</td><td></td><td>OBSERVATION</td></tr>
<tr><td>BREAKFAST</td><td></td></tr>
<tr><td>LUNCH</td><td></td></tr>
<tr><td>DINNER</td><td></td></tr>
<tr><td>SNACKS</td><td></td></tr>
<tr><td>DESSERTS</td><td></td></tr>
</table>

OBSERVATION

INSPIRATION

NOTES & TIPS

DAILY MEAL PLANNER

TO DO	
1	
2	
3	
4	
5	
6	
7	
8	
9	
10	

EXERCISE

GOAL ACTIVITIES

	☐
	☐
	☐
	☐
	☐
	☐
	☐

SHOPPING

<table>
<tr><td colspan="2">MEALS</td></tr>
<tr><td>BREAKFAST</td><td></td></tr>
<tr><td>LUNCH</td><td></td></tr>
<tr><td>DINNER</td><td></td></tr>
<tr><td>SNACKS</td><td></td></tr>
<tr><td>DESSERTS</td><td></td></tr>
</table>

OBSERVATION

INSPIRATION

NOTES & TIPS

DAILY MEAL PLANNER

TO DO	
1	
2	
3	
4	
5	
6	
7	
8	
9	
10	

EXERCISE

GOAL ACTIVITIES

SHOPPING

<table>
<tr><td colspan="2">

MEALS

</td><td>

OBSERVATION

</td></tr>
<tr><td>**BREAKFAST**</td><td></td><td rowspan="3"></td></tr>
<tr><td>**LUNCH**</td><td></td></tr>
<tr><td>**DINNER**</td><td></td></tr>
<tr><td>**SNACKS**</td><td></td><td rowspan="2">

INSPIRATION

</td></tr>
<tr><td>**DESSERTS**</td><td></td></tr>
</table>

NOTES & TIPS